DUKAN BEGINNERS

Learn How to Cook Dukes Diet Food in 90 Minutes and Lose Your Weight

Table of content

Introduction

I want to thank you for purchasing this book, 'Dukan Diet.'

The Dukan diet will help you eat your way to a healthy and a strong body as well as a longer life. The Dukan diet is a low-carb and a high-protein diet. This diet will help you lose weight and maintain the weight loss. Dr. Pierre Dukan, a French General practitioner, is the creator of this amazing diet. The ideology of this diet is quite simple. To lose weight, a person needs to drastically reduce the intake of all foods except proteins.

When you restrict the intake of carbs, the body starts to convert protein and stored fats into glucose through the process of gluconeogenesis. All the fat present in the body is the result of stored glucose. Well, only a portion of the carbs you consume are converted into glucose that is readily used by the body and the rest is stored in the form of fats. When you restrict the intake of fats and carbs, your body's metabolic rate improves, and it helps to support weight loss.

The obvious health benefits include weight loss and the improvement of your heart's health. When you eliminate sugars, fats and starch from your food, your blood sugar levels stabilize. While following this diet, you don't need to count the calories you consume. All that you need to do is ensure that the food you consume is rich in protein and consider minimal carbs. In fact, the only carbs you consume will be in the form of a little oat bran and a small portion of non-starchy vegetables.

There are four stages of this diet. The first phase is the attack phase and it lasts from 5-10 days. During this stage, you need to eliminate all carbs from your diet. The second phase is the cruise phase. In this phase, you can gradually introduce some starchy vegetables. The third phase is the consolidation phase, and in this phase you can include certain food items like dairy and fruit into your diet. The final stage is the stabilization phase. If you notice that any intake of small portions of carbs doesn't lead to weight gain, then you can continue to include such carbs.

Here is a diet that will enable you to eat food that is not only healthy and nutritious, but delicious as well. The Dukan diet is quite unique and you certainly will not disappoint your taste buds with this diet. The recipes that are curated in this book are easy to follow and understand. If you want to step into the world of healthy eating and living, then let us start without further ado.

Chapter One: Dukan Diet Attack Phase Recipes

(Can be used in Cruise phase, Consolidation phase and Stabilization phase)

Scrambled Eggs with Cream Cheese and Chives

Serves: 2

Ingredients:

- 4 egg whites
- 2 whole eggs
- 2 tablespoons fat free cream cheese
- Salt to taste
- Pepper to taste
- 2 tablespoons fresh chives, chopped

Method:

1. Add all the ingredients into a bowl and whisk well.
2. Place a nonstick pan over medium heat. Spray some cooking spray over it. When the pan heats, pour the egg mixture.
3. Stir frequently until the egg cooks as per your liking.

Chicken Tandoori

Serves: 3

Ingredients:

- 3 chicken breasts
- 1 teaspoon tandoori spice blend
- 1 teaspoon ginger, grated
- 1 teaspoon garlic, grated
- 1 jar nonfat yogurt
- 1 chili, minced
- Salt to taste
- Pepper to taste
- 1 tablespoon lemon juice

Method:

1. Place chicken in a bowl.
2. Add rest of the ingredients into a blender and blend until smooth. Pour over the chicken and stir until well coated. Cover and place in the refrigerator for 7-8 hours.
3. Grill on a preheated grill on both the sides until cooked through.
4. Serve hot.

Piri Piri Chicken

Serves: 2

Ingredients:

- 4 chicken thighs or 2 chicken breast fillets, skinless
- 1 clove garlic, finely chopped
- 2 tablespoons cider vinegar
- 1 teaspoon crushed chili flakes
- Salt to taste
- Pepper to taste
- 1 tablespoon lemon juice
- ½ teaspoon paprika
- ½ teaspoon dried oregano

To serve:

- 1 tablespoon lime juice
- Plain nonfat yogurt

Method:

1. Place chicken in a bowl.
2. Add rest of the ingredients except salt and pepper into a bowl and whisk until well combined. Pour over the chicken and stir until well coated. Cover and place in the refrigerator for 7-8 hours.
3. Remove chicken from the marinade and sprinkle salt and pepper over it.
4. Grill on a preheated grill on both the sides until cooked through.
5. Sprinkle lime juice on top and serve with yogurt.

Rosemary Grilled Chicken

Serves: 6

Ingredients:

- 6 chicken breasts (6 ounces each), skinless, boneless
- 8-10 cloves garlic, finely chopped
- 3 teaspoons olive oil
- 1 teaspoon crushed chili flakes
- Salt to taste
- Pepper to taste
- 6 tablespoons lemon juice
- ½ teaspoon smoked paprika
- 3 tablespoons fresh rosemary, minced

Method:

1. Place chicken in a bowl.
2. Add rest of the ingredients into a bowl and whisk until well combined. Pour over the chicken and stir until well coated. Cover and place in the refrigerator for 7-8 hours.
3. Remove chicken from the marinade.
4. Grill on a preheated grill on both the sides until cooked through.

Café Frappe

Serves: 1

Ingredients:

- ½ cup strong black coffee or espresso, cold
- Artificial sweetener of your choice, to taste
- ½ cup skim milk, cold
- Ice cubes, as required

Method:

1. Add all the ingredients into a blender and blend until creamy.
2. Pour into a glass and serve.

Cinnamon Oat Bran Muffins

Serves: 12

Ingredients:

- ¾ cup oat bran
- 4 large eggs
- 2 teaspoons baking powder
- 4 tablespoons cinnamon powder
- 10 tablespoons nonfat plain yogurt
- 2/3 cup splenda

Method:

1. Add oat bran, baking powder, cinnamon powder and splenda into a large bowl and stir.
2. Stir in the eggs and yogurt and whisk until well combined.
3. Grease a 12-count muffin tin with a little butter flavored cooking spray.
4. Pour the batter into the muffin cups. Fill up to 2/3.
5. Bake in a preheated oven at 350° F for 15-18 minutes or a toothpick, when inserted in the center, comes out cool.
6. Remove from the oven and cool for a few minutes. Run a knife around the edges of the muffins. Invert on to a plate and serve.
7. Leftovers can be stored in an airtight container in the refrigerator for 3-4 days.

Pain Doux (French Sweet Bread)

Makes: 1 loaf

Ingredients:

- 8 eggs, separated
- ¾ cup skimmed milk powder
- 2 teaspoons vanilla essence
- A pinch saffron strands
- ½ cup oat bran
- 8-10 tablespoons powdered swerve
- 2 tablespoons baking powder
- A pinch of salt

Method:

1. Add a pinch of salt into the bowl of whites and beat with an electric mixer until stiff.
2. Add yolks and swerve and beat for a couple of minutes.
3. Add oat bran and milk powder and fold gently with a spoon until well combined.
4. Stir in the vanilla, saffron and baking powder.
5. Grease a loaf pan with a little butter flavored cooking spray. Pour the batter in the pan.
6. Bake in a preheated oven at 350° F for 25 minutes. Remove from the oven and cool for a few minutes. Run a knife around the edges of the bread. Invert on to a plate. Slice and serve.
7. Leftovers can be stored in an airtight container in the refrigerator for 3-4 days.

Turkey Burger

Serves: 12

Ingredients:

- 2 1/4 pounds lean minced turkey or beef
- 3-4 egg whites
- Crushed chili to taste
- 6 tablespoons oat bran
- 2 stock cubes, crushed
- Herbs or spices of your choice

Method:

1. Add meat, oat bran and stock cube into a bowl and mix until well combined.
2. Stir in the egg whites and mix until well combined.
3. Add the herbs or spices that you are using. Mix until well combined.
4. Divide the mixture into 12 equal portions and shape into patties.
5. Preheat a grill to medium heat. Grill for 8-10 minutes. Flip sides and grill for 8-10 minutes or until cooked through.
6. Serve.

Italian Flank Steak Pinwheels

Serves: 8

Ingredients:

- 2 teaspoons olive oil
- 2 cloves garlic, minced
- 4 teaspoons curry powder
- 2 pounds lean ground beef or turkey or chicken
- Salt to taste
- Pepper to taste

Method:

1. Place a skillet over medium heat. Add oil. When the oil is heated, stir in the beef and garlic. Cook until brown. Break it simultaneously as it cooks.
2. Stir in the curry powder, pepper and salt.
3. Serve hot.

Baked Vanilla Custard

Serves: 12

Ingredients:

- 10 eggs
- 3 cups skim milk
- ½ cup splenda
- 2 tablespoons vanilla extract
- 2 teaspoons nutmeg

Method:

1. Add eggs into a large bowl and whisk well. Add vanilla, splenda and nutmeg and whisk well.
2. Place a saucepan with milk over low heat. When the mixture is warm, add into the egg mixture beating continuously. Turn off the heat.
3. Pour into 12 ramekins.
4. Place ramekins in a large baking pan. Pour enough water to make a water bath. Place the water bath along with the ramekins into a preheated oven.
5. Bake at 350 °F for 30-40 minutes or until set. Turn off the oven and let the custard cool in the oven for 2 hours.
6. Chill and serve.

Chapter Two: Cruise Phase

(Can be used in Consolidation Phase and Stabilization Phase)

Salmon with Mustard and Dill Sauce

Serves: 2

Ingredients:

- 2 salmon fillets
- ½ tablespoon mustard classic
- 1 tablespoon finely chopped dill
- 1 green onion, chopped
- 3 tablespoons nonfat cottage cheese
- Salt to taste
- Pepper to taste

Method:

1. Place salmon in the freezer for 20-30 minutes.
2. Place salmon on your cutting board. Cut into thin strips.
3. Place a nonstick pan over medium heat. Place salmon strips over it and cook for a minute. Flip sides and cook the other side for a minute. Remove salmon strips and place in a bowl.
4. Place the pan back over heat. Add onion, cottage cheese and mustard and stir. Heat for a minute.
5. Add salmon strips back into the pan. Also add dill, salt and pepper. Mix well.
6. Serve hot.

Meat Loaf

Serves: 5-6

Ingredients:

- 1 pound lean minced beef
- 1 egg, beaten
- 1 hardboiled egg, sliced
- A pinch crushed chili flakes
- 1 teaspoon garlic, minced
- 1 small onion, minced
- 2 tablespoons nonfat fromage frais or yogurt
- Salt to taste
- Pepper to taste

Serving options:

- Herb sauce
- Tomato sauce
- Horseradish sauce

Method:

1. Add egg into a bowl and beat lightly. Add beef, onion, salt, pepper and fromage frais and mix well.
2. Grease lightly a small loaf pan with cooking spray. Add half the meat mixture into the pan. Place egg slices over it. Place the remaining meat mixture over the egg slices and spread it evenly.
3. Bake in a preheated oven at 350 °F for 40-45 minutes or until cooked.
4. Remove from the oven and cool for a few minutes. Slice and serve.
5. Serve with the any of the options mentioned. It can be served hot, warm or cold.

Cheese and Smoked Chicken Casserole

Serves: 2-3

Ingredients:

- 2 cups chopped smoked chicken or shredded roasted chicken
- 2 green onions, thinly sliced
- Salt to taste
- Pepper to taste
- 21 ounces nonfat ricotta cheese or any other creamy cheese
- 2 egg yolks

Method:

1. Add chicken, salt, ricotta cheese, green onion, yolks and pepper into a baking dish.
2. Bake in a preheated oven at 350 °F for 40-45 minutes.
3. Serve hot or warm.

Beef Meatballs with Konjac Rice

Serves: 6

Ingredients:

- 2 pounds ground beef
- 2 small cloves garlic, minced
- Salt to taste
- ½ teaspoon garlic powder
- Pepper to taste
- 1/3 cup mixed flat leaf parsley and dill, chopped
- 2 small onions, finely chopped
- 2 large eggs
- 16 ounces Konjac rice
- 2 green onions, green part only, sliced

Method:

1. Drain Konjac rice in a sieve after rinsing in cold water.
2. Gather all the ingredients and add into a large bowl. Make small balls of the mixture.
3. Place the balls on a lined baking sheet.
4. Bake in a preheated oven at 350 °F for about 20 minutes or until cooked through

Shrimp and Tofu Miso Soup

Serves: 3

Ingredients:

- 3 cups vegetable or chicken broth
- ½ tablespoon ginger, minced
- 2 ½ tablespoons miso
- ¼ teaspoon Asian chili paste
- 1 pound shrimp, peeled
- ¼ cup spring onions, finely chopped
- 2 cups spinach or 2 tablespoons of shredded nori or wakame seaweed
- 2 cups firm silken tofu, cut into 1 inch cubes
- 2 tablespoons soy sauce

Method:

1. Pour broth into a saucepan. Add the seaweeds if using now. Place saucepan over medium heat. Simmer for 5-6 minutes if you like a strong taste. Simmer for lesser time if you like a milder taste.
2. Lower heat. Add miso and little of the hot broth and whisk well. Pour into the saucepan. Add spinach if using now, shrimp, scallions, soy sauce, and tofu.
3. Simmer for a few minutes until the shrimp is cooked.
4. Ladle into soup bowls and serve.

Tofu Shirataki Noodle Soup

Serves: 8

Ingredients:

- 8 cups vegetable stock
- 4 mushrooms, thinly sliced
- 1 pound firm tofu, cubed
- 4 cloves garlic, sliced
- 2 teaspoons ginger, minced
- 7 ounces Shirataki noodles
- 4 scallions or spring onions, roughly sliced
- 4 teaspoons soy sauce
- 2 spring onions or scallions, finely sliced to garnish

Method:

1. Pour vegetable stock into a saucepan. Place the saucepan over medium heat.
2. Add tofu, ginger, and garlic. When it begins to boil, lower the heat and simmer for 5-6 minutes.
3. Add spring onions and soy sauce. Simmer until the noodles are soft.
4. Ladle into soup bowls. Garnish with scallions and serve.

Zucchini Salad

Serves: 2-3

Ingredients:

- 4 zucchinis or courgettes, peeled lengthwise into ribbons
- ¼ cup lemon juice
- ½ teaspoon mustard powder
- A handful fresh basil, torn
- 2 fresh red chilies, chopped
- 2 teaspoons extra-virgin olive oil
- Salt to taste
- 1 cup cherry tomatoes, halved

Method:

1. Add lemon juice, oil, mustard powder and salt into a bowl and whisk well.
2. Place zucchini ribbons in a large bowl. Pour dressing over it. Toss well.
3. Sprinkle basil leaves on top and serve.

Broccoli and Surimi Salad

Serves: 4

Ingredients:

- 2 heads broccoli, cut into bite size pieces
- 10 1/2 ounces fat free yogurt
- 16 surimi sticks, chopped
- 4 teaspoons lemon juice
- Pepper to taste
- Salt to taste

Method:

1. Add broccoli and surimi into a large bowl and toss.
2. Add rest of the ingredients into another bowl and whisk well. Pour over the broccoli and toss well.
3. Chill for 30 minutes and serve.

Scotch Eggs

Serves: 8

Ingredients:

- 10 large eggs
- 4 slices whole meal bread, made into crumbs
- Salad of your choice, to serve
- 16 low fat sausages
- 2 tablespoons oat bran

Method:

1. To make scotch eggs: Boil 8 eggs in a saucepan of boiling water for 8 minutes. Discard the hot water and pour cold water into the pan. Cool for a few minutes. Discard the shells.
2. Discard the casing from the sausages. Take meat from 2 sausages and shape into a ball. Flatten it on your palm. Place a boiled egg on it and enclose the egg by bringing together the edges of the sausages.
3. Repeat with the remaining 8 eggs and sausages.
4. Crack remaining 2 eggs into a shallow bowl and beat well. Place breadcrumbs and oat bran into another shallow bowl.
5. Dip the scotch eggs in the beaten egg. Dredge in breadcrumbs mixture and place on a baking sheet.
6. Bake in a preheated oven at 350 °F for about 20-25 minutes or until golden brown.
7. Cut into 2 halves if desired. Serve with a summer salad if desired.

Lettuce Wraps

Serves: 2-3

Ingredients:

- 7 ounces lean ground beef or steak
- 2 cloves garlic, crushed, minced
- ½ teaspoon onion powder
- ½ teaspoon garlic powder
- A handful fresh cilantro, chopped
- Salt to taste
- Pepper to taste
- 1 small onion, finely minced
- ½ teaspoon dried oregano
- ½ teaspoon cayenne pepper or to taste
- Lettuce leaves, as required

Method:

1. Place a skillet over medium heat. Add beef. Sauté until brown.
2. Stir in onion, garlic powder, onion powder, oregano, cayenne pepper, pepper and a sprinkle of water. Mix well.
3. Lower the heat and simmer for about 10 minutes. Stir frequently. Sprinkle more water if necessary.
4. Add salt and stir.
5. Place the lettuce leaves on a serving platter. Place a little of the beef mixture in each of the lettuce leaves. Serve with tomatoes or Dukan diet friendly salsa.

Chocolate Custard

Serves: 4

Ingredients:

- 4 eggs
- 2 cups skim milk
- 2-3 tablespoons splenda or to taste
- 2 tablespoons reduced fat cocoa powder, unsweetened
- Mint sprigs to garnish

Method:

1. Add eggs into a large bowl and whisk well. Place a saucepan with milk over low heat. When the mixture is warm, add into the egg mixture beating continuously.
2. Cook until the mixture is thick and coats the back of a spoon. Add splenda and whisk well.
3. Cool for a while and pour into 4 wine glasses.
4. Chill and serve.

Spiced Rhubarb Compote with Orange Cream

Serves: 8

Ingredients:

- 3 1/2 ounces fresh root ginger, peeled, grated
- 21 ounces rhubarb, trimmed, cut into 1 cm pieces
- 6 tablespoons low fat crème fraiche
- 6 tablespoons splenda
- 6 tablespoons fat free Greek yogurt
- Zest of 2 oranges, grated
- 10 ounces water

Method:

1. Add water, splenda and ginger into a saucepan. Place the saucepan over medium heat. When it begins to boil, let it simmer for 3-4 minutes.
2. Add rhubarb and stir. Let it simmer for 5 minutes. Turn off the heat and cover with a lid. Set aside to cool. Stir frequently.
3. Add yogurt, zest and crème fraiche into a bowl and beat until well combined.
4. Serve rhubarb in bowls topped with a big blob of orange crème.

Chapter Three: Consolidation Phase

(Can be used in Stabilization phase)

Greek Tzatziki (Appetizer)

Serves: 2-3

Ingredients:

- 1 cucumber, peeled, deseeded, chopped
- 1 small clove garlic, finely minced
- Salt to taste
- White pepper to taste
- 1 tablespoon chopped fresh dill
- 1 cup fat free Greek yogurt

Method:

1. Add yogurt, salt, pepper and garlic into a bowl and mix well.
2. Stir in the cucumber and dill. Cover and refrigerate for 2-3 hours.
3. Serve.

Cheese and Onion Flatbread with Hummus (Appetizer)

Serves: 4

Ingredients:

For flatbread:

- ½ cup oat bran
- 2 eggs, beaten
- 1 3/4 ounces cheddar cheese, grated
- 6 tablespoons fat free natural yogurt
- 4 spring onions, finely chopped
- A few drops of oil to fry

For hummus:

- 2 cans (14.5 ounces each) chickpeas, drained, rinsed
- ¼ cup fat free natural yogurt
- Juice of a lemon
- Salt to taste
- Pepper to taste
- 2 cloves garlic, peeled
- ½ cup fresh parsley, chopped
- ¼ teaspoon paprika
- Water, as required

Method:

1. To make hummus: Add all the ingredients of hummus into a blender and blend until the texture you desire is achieved.
2. Transfer into a bowl. Cover and set aside for a while for the flavors to set in.

3. To make flatbread: Add oat bran, eggs, cheese, yogurt and spring onions into a bowl and whisk well.
4. Place a nonstick pan over medium heat. Add 3 drops oil into the pan. Swirl the pan and wipe the pan with paper towels.
5. Spread half the mixture on the pan (in the center of the pan). Cook until it gets golden brown on both sides. Chop into wedges.
6. Serve wedges with hummus.

Haricot Beans, Tuna and Mint Pate (Appetizer)

Serves: 8

Ingredients:

- 2 cans (14.5 ounces each) haricot beans, drained, rinsed
- 2 cans (4.5 ounces each) tuna in spring water
- Juice of a lemon
- 2 tablespoons fresh mint leaves, chopped
- 2 tablespoons fat free Greek yogurt
- 1 red bell pepper, deseeded, sliced
- 1 yellow bell pepper, deseeded, sliced

Method:

1. Add haricot beans, 1 can tuna, lemon juice, salt, pepper and yogurt into a blender and blend until it is almost smooth.
2. Transfer into a bowl. Add 1 can tuna and mint and stir.
3. Dip bell peppers in haricot beans mixture and enjoy.

Stuffed Eggs with Shrimps/Prawns (Appetizer)

Serves: 12 (2 halves per serving)

Ingredients:

- 12 hard-boiled eggs, peeled, halved lengthwise
- 3-4 tablespoons Dukan friendly oil free mayonnaise
- 1 pound shrimp / prawn, rinsed, cleaned, cooked, finely chopped
- Paprika to garnish

Method:

1. Carefully scoop out the yolks and add into a bowl. Mash the yolks.
2. Add mayonnaise and shrimp and mix well.
3. Fill this mixture into the cavities of the yolks in the egg halves.
4. Sprinkle paprika on top and serve.

Pancakes

Serves: 2

Ingredients:

- 4 tablespoons oat bran
- 3 tablespoons fat free fromage frais
- 2 tablespoons wheat bran
- 1 large egg, beaten
- 3-4 teaspoons skim milk
- Herbs of your choice
- Salt to taste
- Pepper powder to taste
- ¼ teaspoon garlic powder
- Sweetener to taste (optional, to be used if you prefer sweet pancakes)

For toppings: Optional, use as required

- Flaked tuna
- Smoked salmon
- Extra lean ham (optional)
- Nuts etc.

Method:

1. Mix together in a bowl, oat bran, fromage frais, wheat bran, herbs, salt, and pepper. Add the beaten egg.
2. Spray a nonstick pan with cooking spray. Pour half the batter.
3. Cook until the bottom side is golden brown. Flip sides and cook the other side too.
4. Repeat the above 2 steps to make the other pancake.
5. Place toppings over it and serve.

Dukan Pizza

Serves: 8

Ingredients:

- 8 cherry tomatoes, sliced
- ¼ cup fat free yogurt
- 4 button mushrooms, sliced
- 2 tablespoons low fat cheese
- 2 teaspoons baking powder
- 4 tablespoons oat bran
- ¼ cup red pepper, diced
- 4 eggs, beaten
- 2 tablespoons corn flour
- 2 chicken breast pieces, pre-cooked, cut into pieces
- Basil leaves, torn to garnish

Method:

1. Add eggs, yogurt, oat bran, basil, corn flour, baking powder and half the chicken pieces into a bowl and mix well.
2. Place a nonstick pan over medium heat. Add remaining chicken pieces. Cook until they are golden brown and crisp.
3. Lower the heat. Pour the egg mixture over the chicken pieces. Cover the pan. Cook for a while until the base is done.
4. Sprinkle tomatoes, bell pepper, mushrooms and cheese on top. Cook until the cheese melts. Grill for a few minutes if desired.
5. Cut into wedges and serve.

Crab Burgers

Serves: 8

Ingredients:

- 2 pounds crab meat
- 8 spring onions, finely chopped
- Zest of 2 lemons, grated
- Juice of 2 lemons
- 4 eggs, beaten
- 7 ounces breadcrumbs
- 1 3/4 ounce mangetout, shredded
- 4 red peppers, deseeded, thinly sliced
- 4 tablespoons sesame seeds, toasted
- ¼ cup fresh parsley, chopped
- ½ Chinese cabbages, shredded
- 24 cherry tomatoes, halved
- 2 teaspoons olive oil
- Salt to taste
- Pepper to taste

Method:

1. Add crabmeat, spring onions, eggs, parsley, zest, breadcrumbs, salt and pepper into a bowl and mix well.
2. Divide the mixture into 8 equal portions. Moisten your hands and shape each portion into a patty.
3. Place a nonstick pan over medium heat. Add 3 drops oil into the pan. Swirl the pan and wipe the pan with paper towels.
4. Place 3-4 burgers on the pan. Cook until it gets golden brown on both sides. Cook the remaining burgers in batches.

5. Add cabbage, tomatoes, mangetout and red peppers into a bowl and toss well.
6. Drizzle olive oil and lemon juice and toss again.
7. Divide the salad into 8 plates. Place a burger on each plate. Sprinkle sesame seeds and serve.

Shrimp Shirataki Diablo

Serves: 2

Ingredients:

- 2 cups cooked or uncooked thawed shrimp
- 1 cup organic corn
- 1 cup peas
- 2 teaspoons dried oregano
- 2 teaspoons red pepper flakes
- 2 cloves garlic, minced
- Salt to taste
- Pepper to taste
- 2/3 cup Dukan diet friendly marinara sauce
- A handful fresh cilantro, chopped, to garnish
- 2 teaspoons dried basil
- 1 teaspoon chipotle chili powder
- 2 teaspoons olive oil or grape seed oil
- 2 packages Shirataki noodles

Method:

1. Place a pan over medium heat. Add oil. When the oil is heated, add garlic and sauté until fragrant. Stir in the shrimp and sauté until light pink.
2. Stir in the corn, peas, pepper, oregano, basil, red pepper flakes and chipotle chili powder. Mix well.
3. Add marinara sauce and mix well.
4. Stir in the Shirataki noodles and mix well. Heat thoroughly.
5. Sprinkle cilantro on top and serve.

Cinnamon & Caramel Cheesecake

Serves: 8-10

Ingredients:

- 2 1/4 pounds Philadelphia cheese or any other low fat soft cheese
- 4 eggs
- 4 tablespoons cornstarch
- 2 teaspoons cinnamon powder
- 10 1/2 ounces nonfat Greek yogurt or low fat sour cream
- 8-10 tablespoons sweetener
- 2 teaspoons sugar free caramel sauce or caramel essence

Method:

1. Add cheese, yogurt, sweetener, eggs and cornstarch into a bowl and whisk well.
2. Stir in the caramel sauce and cinnamon.
3. Pour into a baking dish.
4. Bake in a preheated oven at 350 °F for about 40-45 minutes or until set.
5. Cool completely and chill for a few hours.
6. Slice and serve.

Chapter Four: Stabilization Phase

Mini Mushroom Frittatas

Serves: 6

Ingredients:

- ½ tablespoon butter
- ¼ teaspoon fresh thyme leaves, finely chopped
- 2 ounces reduced fat Swiss cheese
- 4 egg whites
- 2 whole eggs
- 1 tablespoon skim milk
- ½ teaspoon salt or to taste
- Pepper powder to taste
- 1 small onion, thinly sliced
- 4 ounces crimini mushrooms, sliced
- ¼ teaspoon Worcestershire sauce

Method:

1. Place a pan over low heat. Add butter. When butter melts, add onions and sauté until golden brown. Stir occasionally.
2. Add thyme, salt and pepper. Remove the onions with a slotted spoon and set aside.
3. Add mushrooms into the same pan. Sauté until tender. Add salt and pepper. If you find that the mushrooms are burning, spray a little cooking spray. Turn off the heat. Add the onions back into the pan and stir.
4. Add eggs, egg whites, salt, Worcestershire sauce and milk into a bowl and whisk until well combined.
5. Add cheese and stir.

6. Grease a 6-count muffin tin with cooking spray. Divide and place the mushrooms into the muffin cups.
7. Divide and pour the egg mixture over the mushrooms. Stir lightly.
8. Bake in a preheated oven at 350 °F for about 15 minutes or until set.
9. Cool for a while. Run a knife around the edges of the frittata. Invert on to a plate
10. Serve warm or cold.

Chicken Korma

Serves: 2

Ingredients:

- 1 medium onion, finely chopped
- ½ tablespoon mustard
- ½ teaspoon garam masala powder
- 2 tablespoons fresh cilantro, chopped to serve
- 3 1/2 ounces virtually fat free quark
- 2 ¾ ounces fat free natural yogurt
- 10 1/2 ounces chicken breasts, cut into strips
- 1 tablespoon lemon juice

Method:

1. Whisk together in a bowl, onion, quark, and mustard until well combined.
2. Add yogurt and garam masala and stir. Add chicken. Mix until the chicken is well coated.
3. Cover and refrigerate for 6-8 hours.
4. Transfer the chicken along with the marinade into a baking dish.
5. Bake in a preheated oven at 400 °F for about 20-30 minutes or until the chicken is cooked. Stir the chicken a couple of times while it is baking.
6. Sprinkle lemon juice and cilantro. Serve hot.

Chicken and Herb Omelet Sandwich

Serves: 2

Ingredients:

- 2 tablespoons wheat bran
- 4 tablespoons wheat bran
- 2 teaspoons baking powder
- 2 egg whites
- 4 whole eggs
- ¼ cup fromage frais
- 2 tablespoons parsley, chopped
- 3 1/2 ounces cooked chicken breast
- 2 tablespoons quark
- Herbs of your choice, minced
- Few drops of olive oil

Method:

1. Add oat bran, wheat bran, baking powder, 2 whole eggs, herbs and fromage frais into a rectangular microwave safe bowl.
2. Microwave on High for 4 minutes.
3. Remove from the microwave and let it cool for a while. Cut into 4 equal slices.
4. Toast the slices lightly.
5. Whisk together in a bowl, 2 eggs, egg whites and some herbs.
8. Place a nonstick pan over medium heat. Add 3 drops oil into the pan. Swirl the pan and wipe the pan with paper towels.
6. Pour half the egg mixture and make an omelet.
7. Repeat the above 2 steps to make the other omelet.
8. Spread ½ tablespoon quark on each of the bread slices.

9. Place 2 bread slices on your cutting board. Divide the chicken pieces over the bread slices. Place an omelet over each bread.
10. Cover with the remaining 2 bread slices. Cut into desired shapes.
11. Serve.

Bacon Omelet

Serves: 1

Ingredients:

- 2 rashers fat reduced bacon, cut into thin strips
- 1 3/4 ounces skimmed milk
- A little fresh parsley, finely chopped
- 2 eggs, beaten
- 1 clove garlic, minced
- Pepper to taste

Method:

1. Add all the ingredients except bacon into a bowl. Whisk well.
2. Add bacon and stir.
3. Place a nonstick frying pan over medium heat. Add the egg mixture and cook until set.
4. Carefully slide on to a plate and serve.

Conclusion

I want to thank you once again for purchasing this book.

Weight loss might be difficult to achieve and even trickier to maintain. However, with the low-carb and high-protein Dukan diet, you can turn your life around.

The recipes that are mentioned in this book are not only easy to understand but are quite simple to follow as well. If you follow these recipes, you will be able to whip up delicious and tasty food within no time! So, all that you need to do is stock up your pantry with the necessary ingredients and get cooking.

Thank you and all the best!

Made in the USA
Middletown, DE
22 March 2021

Made in the USA
Coppell, TX
07 August 2020